HEARING AIDS
HOW TO SUCCESSFULLY WEAR HEARING AIDS

Chris Scire

http://www.cshaa.co.uk

Publishers Information

Copyright © 2014 Chris Scire

This edition published in 2014 by Kindle Publishers Pathway

ISBN- 13:978-1499201383
ISBN-10:1499201389

TABLE OF CONTENTS

CHAPTER 1.

WHY I WROTE THIS BOOK

I wrote this book to share some simple strategies to enable someone to achieve success with their hearing aid. Most people are surprised at how many factors are involved in providing them with the right hearing aid solution.

People who buy hearing aids have genuine concerns and they want to get it right and know that their investment was a good one.

They are concerned that it will be visible and people will know they have a hearing loss.

They are concerned about whether they can handle it or not. They are concerned about whether the benefit of the aid will justify the cost involved.

And they are concerned that it will not work well and leave them disappointed.

It is hoped that by producing this guide, these and other concerns can be addressed and overcome.

What is encouraging, is that today, more options are available than ever to help the patient find acceptance of a hearing aid solution that is personal to them. It is not necessarily buying the best hearing aid on the market but of buying a hearing aid that the patient is willing to wear. This is certainly the best hearing aid money can buy.

CHAPTER 2.

WHY YOU SHOULD READ THIS BOOK

This book will help you to overcome the barriers that are there that hinder hearing aid success. There are so many documented benefits to wearing hearing aids that it seems a shame that so many of them end up in the drawer. This includes both NHS as well as private hearing aids if the truth be told.

I have met many a private patient who has come to my clinic who simply doesn't wear their hearing aid any more. This is generally due to various unresolved issues with the performance of the hearing aid and of the hearing aid retailer.

If with the right attitude and support the patient can overcome these barriers then a new quality of life is waiting to be accessed that can transform lives of both the individual and loved ones.

If you are such a person who has encountered a barrier to better hearing then I would like to encourage you to pick up where you left off.

Read the chapters, renew your determination, and overcome whatever the issue is and enjoy better hearing.

CHAPTER 3.

Accept It - You Have A Hearing Loss

This is perhaps the hardest step of all. But once taken, it is life changing. If you have not accepted it either, then let me encourage you. The earlier that you can accept it, the easier and sooner you will enjoy the benefits of better hearing.

Having a hearing loss has a massive effect on an individual in many ways. Not just socially but psychologically, physically as well as emotionally.

Everyone suffers in some way from the psychological effects of a hearing loss and experiences a sense of grief. These stages of grief have to be worked through before the person reaches a place of acceptance.

Such is the prevailing stigma associated with having a hearing loss that most people take on average between seven to ten years to do something about it from the onset of symptoms.

It still surprises me even now, just how many things people will say to deny they have a loss.

Some of these excuses are; people don't talk properly today, everyone mumbles, the television isn't as good as it used to be and my spouse is softly spoken.

No matter how hard a person in a group conversation with a hearing loss tries to bluff, nod and smile, they still cannot follow the conversation in a noisy environment. It just leads to miserable social isolation.

There are millions of people in the world who have a hearing loss. So if you have a hearing loss, you are not alone.

At the current rate, it is estimated that by 2030, 1 in 4 of the population will have some form of hearing loss.

A concern for some people is about what other people might think about them. If you think about it, probably all the people they know in their life, know they have a hearing loss. As often is the case, the last person to realise is the person with the hearing loss.

It may not be easy. Embarrassment and denial have to be dealt with.

It may not be pleasant to acknowledge the effects of the hearing loss , but it is an important step in the process to finding a solution.

Once you are at the place of acceptance, the journey to better hearing can begin.

CHAPTER 4.

Two Really Is Better Than One.

Can I get away with only having one? This is a frequent question from some people when they come for a hearing test. It is my own opinion that if the patient has a hearing loss in both ears that can be aided then inmost cases they need two hearing aids. The word binaural is made up of "bi" for two and "aural" for ears. It has been demonstrated by binaural hearing aid wearers that they have a better listening experience than monaural wearers.

The top ten reasons for wearing two hearing aids are as follows:

1.One is half a system.

One ear working less effectively can have a significant impact on the wearers daily life. It is like closing one eye. You can still see but it is less effective.

2.Improvement in localisation.

This is simply that balanced hearing improves our ability to pin point and locate which direction the sound source is coming from.

3.The bigger picture.

We actually hear in the brain and not in the ears. Taking input from both ears means that the brain's natural signal processor enables these input sounds to be blended together into a single coherent sound picture.

4. Stereo balance is important.

In order to enjoy true sound perception,it is necessary for both ears to receive evenly. Without such equality the brain is presented with incomplete information.

5.Reduction in Noise.

Both ears work together effectively to enable the brain to locate and isolate one sound over another depending on the interest value of the sound signal. This filtering and reduction of background noise is one of the best reasons to wear two hearing aids.

6.Selective hearing.

Because of the dampening down of noise the brain is able to therefore focus on certain sounds that you might want to listen to. This means that depending on the nature of the hearing loss, the patient might not have to work as hard to hear effectively in certain listening environments.

7.A more natural sound quality.

When both ears are working together a richer, smoother sound quality is experienced.

8.Stress free and relaxed hearing.

When both ears are working together, it takes less work and stress to hear correctly. I have often experienced this when fitting a hearing aid system. Once the aids are worn, the straining and effort goes and the patients face relaxes.

9.Complete peace of mind.

Two hearing aids means that less amplification is needed to achieve a comfortable listening experience. There is also the peace of mind gained by knowing that the unaided ear is not suffering auditory deterioration at a faster rate than the aided ear. Stimulation of the hearing nerves by the hearing aids can slow down the rate of deterioration.

10.Increased confidence.

Hearing on both sides means that the patient can respond accurately and without hesitation. This boosts confidence and self-esteem. So no matter where the conversation takes place, the hearing aid wearer is socially connected to the conversation.

CHAPTER 5.

A Thorough Hearing Consultation

It is vital for a thorough and proper consultation to be carried out to assess the nature and type of your hearing loss. This should be carried out by a suitably qualified and registered hearing aid audiologist. During the consultation several different tests should be carried out.

The main components of the hearing test consultation are as follows:

CASE HISTORY

The hearing test usually begins with a detailed conversation about your hearing problems and experiences. This should include questions about past medical history, exposure to excessive noise and hearing issues affecting your lifestyle. This enables the hearing aid audiologist to determine the extent and nature of the hearing loss. It also ensures that a referral to a GP does not have to take place.

OTOSCOPY

This is when the hearing aid audiologist will examine the ear with an otoscope. It is quite painless. This is to check that there is no physical damage or abnormalities causing the hearing loss and to make sure that the canal is free of wax . Wax is a common cause of hearing problems. By inspecting the outer ear, ear canal and ear drum, the hearing aid audiologist is making sure that each part is healthy and that it would be safe to take an accurate impression of the ear canal if required.

UNAIDED SPEECH TEST

With this test, you listen to a list of words spoken at different volumes and then you have to repeat back what you have heard. This test shows how well you hear speech and conversations.

AUDIOMETRY

This is the main part of the hearing consultation. You enter a soundproof test booth, put on some headphones and press a response button every time you hear a beep or a buzz. The procedure must conform to the agreed BSA regulations. The test results are recorded on a graph called an audiogram.

EXPLANATION OF RESULTS

After obtaining reliable results, the hearing aid audiologist then goes on to explain your hearing loss and prescription. It is important that you understand the explanation of what is happening to your hearing and why. This helps you to move forward and to take the necessary steps to overcome your hearing problem.

GIVEN A DEMONSTRATION OF BENEFIT

If you do require hearing aids, the hearing aid audiologist should give you a demonstration of the benefit of hearing aids. Test hearing aids are generally used.

SHOWN ALTERNATIVES

Make sure that you are shown all the alternatives that are available for your hearing loss,including all the facts needed to enable you to make an informed decision. You should also be free from any sales pressure. If it is experienced, remember you do not have to make a decision there and then.

CHAPTER 6.

Use An Independent

By using an independent hearing aid audiologist you will generally get someone who runs their own practice. This means it is even more important for them to deliver a high standard of personal service, as satisfied patients are the life blood of their business. Most of which comes from personal recommendations.

This also means that you benefit from continuity of service and get to know your hearing aid audiologist. They will understand your needs better. This is something you don't always get with a national company. It is common for hearing aid dispensers to move around from one company to another looking for a better package.

Because they are independent, they are not tied to one particular manufacturer and so can offer the widest choice available of suitable hearing aid solutions.

Most independents actually care for their patients because they have a genuine desire to make a difference and to change lives through hearing aid provision.

My aim as an independent has always been to do my best to provide my patients with professional personal patient centred hearing healthcare.

CHAPTER 7.

The Benefits Of Open Fit

The Open fit hearing aid is a relatively new hearing aid style. They have been well received by the consumer and have really grown in popularity since they were launched. They are generally small, very light and discreet devices that are set up behind or just on top of the ear. This type of hearing aid comes in two models, the Acoustic thin tube model or the Receiver in the ear model.

The difference between the two models is that in the Acoustic tube model, all the components are in the hearing aid casing. As compared to the Receiver in the ear model, where all the components are contained in the hearing aid casing with the receiver being placed in the ear canal. This has the advantage of providing a better signal quality as well as allowing for greater amplification.

In my experience, acceptance to wearing Open fit hearing aids is high due to the following reasons.

1.This style is great for diminishing the occlusion effect. The feeling of being block up.

2.They are generally light, small and easy for the patient to fit.

3.They are great for those who have a high frequency hearing loss but also have normal low frequencies.

4.They have well positioned automatic directional microphones. This helps to provide the wearer with better speech understanding in the presence of background noise.

5. They are affordable in the lower technology levels.

CHAPTER 8.

Apply The Three Month Rule

Wearing hearing aids is not a quick fix. This may comes as a surprise to you but it is not as easy as say wearing a pair of glasses. The process of adaptation is much more complicated.

The brain needs time in order to relearn how to hear and to cope with the processing of all the new sounds. Your hearing if it is an age related hearing loss, developed gradually over many years. Likewise the brain needs time to gradually get use to amplified sound again. Research has shown that it takes the brain between one to three months for the brain to adapt to normal hearing levels.

Many people have missed out on the benefits of wearing hearing aids simply because they gave up too soon.

I recommend and supply to my patients a guided rehabilitation plan to follow that eases them into wearing the hearing aids.

Put simply, start gradually,be patient and persevere. You will hit problems that need to be worked through. Expect to go through a period of adjustment. The hearing aids will probably need to be fine tuned as your brain adapts to the new sounds, so expect to have a series of follow up appointments. You also have to adjust to listening again and this applies to your family and friends.

It helps to be realistic as well. If you have hearing nerve damage, you are not going to get back perfect hearing and hear well all the time. Even people with normal hearing levels struggle to hear in certain environments.

You will be able to get used to all these adjustments. It also helps to use hearing tactics to improve communication. Hearing tactics are strategies that are put in place to help the wearer to communicate as best they can in the sound environments they find themselves in. An example of this would be taking control of the room. You decide where to sit. Don't allow someone to sit you somewhere in the room where you cannot hear.

CHAPTER 9.

You Must Have This Technology

Do the best that you can for your hearing. Work out your budget and get the best hearing aid technology that you can afford. Aim to get the best value for your money.

This can be accomplished by ensuring that you are buying the latest technology from the retailer. Some companies re-brand their hearing aids so that it is difficult to know who the manufacturer is and what the level of technology is being bought. Make sure you find out so that you do not purchase older technology.

Your aim should be to for the hearing aid to have at least the following technology :

1.Feedback Management.

This technology will ensure that your hearing aid doesn't produce that annoying and embarrassing whistling of the hearing aid.

2.Noise Reduction.

This technology will reduce unwanted background noise and provided a comfortable listening experience.

3.Speech Enhancement.

These systems within a hearing aid enhance the speech component of the sound signal.

4.Directional Microphones.

This feature helps to combine some of the above technology to further improve the signal to noise ratio so that speech clarity is achieved even in the presence of background noise.

CHAPTER 10.

Keep Positive And Be Determined

Having a positive attitude is everything. It can be the deciding factor between success and failure.

I have seen first hand with my own patients the results of having a positive attitude and its relationship to their being a successful outcome.

The patient who has a "can do" approach, overcomes the various problems that can occur as the hearing aids are personalised to their hearing prescription. They appreciate that it takes time for the brain to adapt and they exercise patience as well as determination. They have a sense of humour and don't worry if they make a mistake. They don't give up. They try again. They are willing to try new things and to approach things in different ways.

When they start to experience the joy of better hearing and start to join in and participate in conversations again, they exhibit a sense of pride in their accomplishment. It is a joy to look back on their journey to see where they started and to see their progress to better hearing. To them it is all worth it. On the other hand, I have had patients who have not had a positive attitude and instead just make excuses and are not even willing to try to get use to a new hearing aid no matter how much you try as a professional to help them.

The ones who are the most successful, are generally the patients who just don't give in and persevere.

CHAPTER 11.

Fit For Purpose

It is difficult to maintain a positive attitude if there are genuine problems with the hearing aid and the fitting. Getting use to amplified sound is one thing, dealing with a problem hearing aid and fitting is another.

You must not just leave a problem if there is one with the hearing aid or fitting. You must make sure it gets sorted out by the hearing aid professional.

I have met several people who have just given up at the first sign of a problem. They just stopped wearing the hearing aid. They did not even tell the dispenser there was a problem and admitted that it was a complete waste of their money.

If only people would go back to the hearing aid audiologist and tell them there is a problem. The vast majority of user problems are quite easy and simple to sort out.

Again, it comes back to persevering until there is a satisfactory outcome and not giving up until the hearing aid is fit for purpose.

If the In-The-Ear hearing aid doesn't fit, it can be re-made. If the In-The-Ear causes any pain because it is too tight, it can be reduced. The microphone and receiver can be replaced if they fail. The battery door can be replaced if it gets broken off. In fact, most things that can go wrong can be dealt with.

So, make sure the aid is fit for purpose and don't give up until you are satisfied with it.

CHAPTER 12.

Some Helpful Features

It is worth considering whether or not you need some additional help when it comes to using and handling the hearing aids.

Even with the best hearing aids, I have found that my patients have benefitted from these options.

1.Have a volume control.

Some patients benefit from having manual control of the volume. This could be by using a remote control or having one fitted to the hearing aid. Sound levels are subjective and there can be a difference between what the hearing aid delivers in terms of amplification and the actual level you need to hear with. This can help you in a very practical way to adjust to new sounds as well as amplified sound.

2.Add an air vent.

This mainly applies to custom made hearing aids. It can really help to overcome that "plugged up" feeling when wearing a custom hearing aid to add a vent. This enables the hearing aid to have a more natural sound and the flow of air can help ease any discomfort caused by the seal of the hearing aid creating a suction effect on the ear drum. The vent also helps to reduce the build up of moisture which can cause a hearing aid to stop working.

3.Use assistive devices.

Check that the hearing aid is compatible for telephone use. Can it be used with a loop system or an FM system? There are quite a few hearing aids on the market now that have a wide range of bluetooth and wireless accessories which connect the wearer to the TV, mobile, MP3's and PC to name a few.

CHAPTER 13.

The Magic Of Marketing

It is sometimes difficult to be realistic when it comes to expectations of a new hearing aid system. Whenever a new product is launched, it is promoted with marketing that has to justify why the hearing aid is so much better than the previous model.

One of my patients read the website of a manufacturer's new hearing aid and was left thinking that all his hearing problems were over.

If the claims of a manufacturer are to be believed as advertised they should support those claims with independent research. No matter what the hearing aid, even if it claims to be the best one, has advantages and disadvantages.

There are many variables involved in order to achieve a successful outcome of better hearing. No matter how good it is claimed to be, success is not just down to the hearing aid system.

You still have to be realistic. With a correctly

fitted prescribed hearing aid you will notice improvements in your hearing but that doesn't mean you will hear everything you want to in every situation.

A hearing aid is just that. An aid to help you hear better. It cannot restore the effects of hearing nerve damage. You will be successful with wearing your hearing aids, if you can be realistic with your expectations of what the hearing aid can and can't do.

CHAPTER 14.

Your Summary Checklist

I hope you have found these strategies useful and that they help you to be successful in wearing your hearing aids. Below is a checklist to ensure that you have considered each one.

1. Accept that you have a hearing loss.

2. Consider wearing two hearing aids.

3. Make sure you have a thorough hearing test consultation.

4. Use an independent hearing aid audiologist.

5. Try wearing an open fit solution.

6. Apply the three month rule.

7. Have a minimum level of technology.

8. Keep positive and be determined.

9. Make sure the hearing aid is fit for purpose.

10. Consider the useful features.

11. Be realistic with marketing claims.

12.Use the checklist.

CHAPTER 15.

A Fantastic Offer!

I hope that you have found this guide useful and as a thank you for reading it, I want to make you a very special , limited offer.

Save £100's Even £1000's

A Fantastic 67% Off

High Street Prices

Applies To

5* & 4* Rated Hearing Aids

As Stated In My Hearing Aid Prices Guide

With This Coupon*

*Terms and Conditions apply

1.Only one voucher per person.
2.Please quote the coupon code HAP2
3.The hearing test fee is a non-refundable £25.
4.This offer is subject to change at any time.

CHAPTER 16.

ABOUT THE AUTHOR

My name is Chris Scire, and for the past 10 years I have been a professionally qualified registered hearing aid audiologist.This includes being a Fellow of the British Society of Hearing Aid Audiologists and registered with the Health Care Professions Council.Over those years I have built up a good reputation within the industry. I was very successful as a branch manager with a national company before setting up my own practice. I was a finalist in the "Audiologist Of The Year 2012" competition out of over 500 UK audiologists.

I have met many people from all walks of life over the years and have experience in dealing with people's problems and frustrations. My philosophy is patient centred dispensing. This is carried out in a friendly personal consultative style, where nothing is too much trouble. I don't use sales tactics to sell you the most expensive hearing aids.

If you have a question or just want a friendly chat, just contact me at chris@cshaa.co.uk

I look forward to hearing from you.

Kind regards

Chris

Rev Chris Sciré BA PGCE DIPTH RHAD FSHAA

CHAPTER 17.

OTHER BOOKS BY CHRIS SCIRE

Hearing Aid Prices Guide 2014

UK Kindle Edition

http://www.amazon.co.uk/HEARING-AID-PRICES-GUIDE-2014-ebook/dp/B00JAJGFSI

USA Kindle Edition

http://www.amazon.com/HEARING-AID-PRICES-GUIDE-2014-ebook/dp/B00JAJGFSI

One Last Thing...

If you enjoyed this book or found it useful, I would appreciate it if you would post a short review on Amazon. Your support really does make a difference and I read all the reviews personally so I can get your feedback and make this book even better.

If you would like to leave a review then all you need to do is visit the review link on Amazon here:

In the UK

http://www.amazon.co.uk/gp/product/B00JSR3CLA

In the US

http://www.amazon.com/gp/product/B00JSR3CLA

Thanks again for your support!

DISCLAIMER

The End

www.ingramcontent.com/pod-product-compliance
Lightning Source LLC
Chambersburg PA
CBHW070720180526
45167CB00004B/1551